Essential Oils
50 Spring Diffuser Recipes and Blends

Table of content

Introduction

Well, whether you're planning to read this post that's important to know. It is amazing. It is fantastic. It'll change your life. Diffusing is not only a way or a chemical free air freshener to help purify the air, but it does lots of other things like helping boost energy, to alter mood, or change your mindset. It may also help to improve typical pressure or daily "moods" or improve concentration or focus. Citrus Essential Oils are a favorite of mine throughout the year. With their scent that is uplifting and energizing, you'll surely find on approaching wet spring days, me reaching for them. Below is a listing of essential oils chosen for springtime use at heart. This is a highly subjective list and is meant solely as a starting point to your investigation.

Whether you are looking for a few thoughts that are new or just are not sure what to do with all of these essential oils in your cupboard, we've got you covered. This is a set of 50 wonderful essential oil recipes for your diffuser, gathered from around the web.

Throughout the springtime, it's fine to savor fresh, clean fragrances that help to market clarity and cleanliness. Here is a wonderful DIY essential oil recipe this month to diffuse around the house. Utilize a blend of Lemon, Pine and Sweet Orange essential oils quantified out to approximately 15 ml. There doesn't must be an exact measurement for diffusing oils, so we advocate using your smell preferences to determine which essential oil you'd like to stand out most in the mix.

Here are a small number of things to notice before you start diffusing.

You require a cool-air diffuser. These diffusers normally require a little bit of distilled water to be added together with essential oils. When you're attempting to diffuse your living room and bedroom, most likely you'll need two diffusers. This one is my favorite for the money and size/features.

You want essential oils. (If you're new to essential oils, here is how I use them in my everyday life.) Some recipes have several variations. Feel free to test to find the one that works for you. Essential Oils bring their curative advantages to the body as they can be absorbed into the blood stream via the skin or lungs. The aromatic aromas can have a gratifying and powerful effect on our general wellbeing. As the Essential Oils enter the bloodstream, they take their curative powers to the part of the body that is in most need.

With First Aid and Common Ailments, you will find over a period you will make up more products which you use frequently, and this will bring even more advantages to you and your family.

For small areas a couple of drops of Lavender (tidy) directly from the bottle, onto region followed by ice pack is perfect. For large regions use fusion above (I have this made up in refrigerator consistently) as it is even better if Aloe Vera Gel mixture is cold.

Creating a mixture of Essential Oils offers you a synergy of the oils. That means the combined advantage of the oils is higher than its individual oils. Recall your 100% Essential Oil mix is not for use in your body it must be a diluted combination for body usage.

The recipe offers you great oil; use this should you prefer to use body oil, instead of a moisturizer creme. The body is very good to give supple skin look and ideal for dry skin or skin in harsh climates where even the most wonderful of skin has a tendency to dry up. Apply all over the body, for added directly to a bath with skin remains moist and gently pat dry.

Your "crowning glory" is an essential section of your look and your self-assurance. In case, your hair is oily, messy or lifeless it doesn't matter how nicely you dress your appearance lacks the finesse of the 'jointly' look. Why do you think there is the term 'bad hair day'?

Chapter 1 – Spring Diffuser Recipes and Blends 1 to 10

1. Essential Oil Combinations for Mental Clarity

Mix oils like Lemon, Peppermint, Hyssop and Rosemary in these five diffuser combinations by Aroma Web to boost concentration and memory.

In her post 10 Must-Try Essential Oil Recipes for Your Diffuser, Jill of The Prairie Homestead recommends a mixture of two drops each of Wild Orange and Peppermint essential oils "to raise alertness, or when you need a fast pick-me-up."

"This treatment works well in case you can have the diffuser near your head while it is being used."

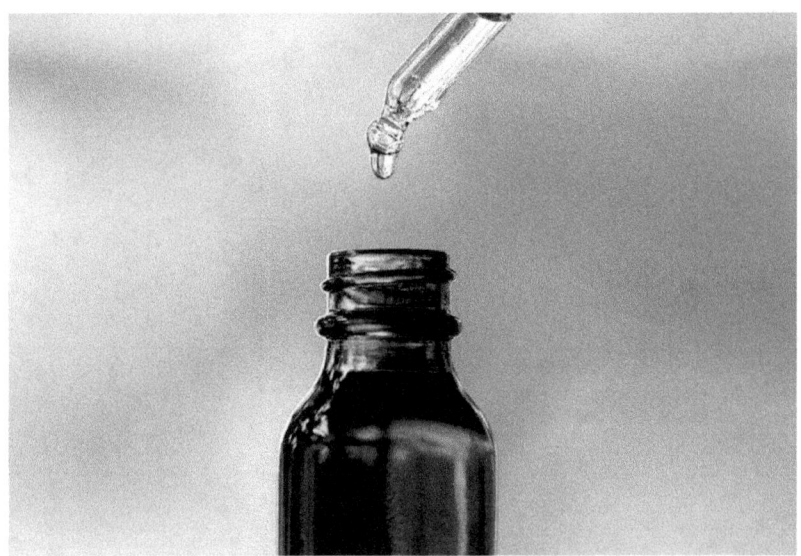

Try this Focus Blend from Laura on Green Living Ladies by combining 2 drops Frankincense, two drops Vetiver, and four drops of a synergy combination like Eden's Garden Align or do TERRA Equilibrium in your diffuser.

2. Energizing Essential Oil Combinations

Combine earthy oils like Frankincense and Ginger with strong green herbs like Basil, Peppermint, and Rosemary in these 4 diffuser fusion from Aroma Web to increase your energy levels around your house or at the office.

Laura of Green Living Women offers her Energizing Blend combining 4 drops each of Peppermint and Wild Orange essential oils.

Laura additionally advocates for Work Out Time, diffusing 2 drops each of Peppermint and Grapefruit essential oils with 2 drops of do TERRA Slim & Sassy metabolic mixture to boost vigor and performance.

3. Essential Oil Blends for Sensuality

To set the perfect mood for a romantic meeting, try this Sweetly Sensual Diffuser Incorporation from Simple Aromatherapy Recipes. Combine 7 – 10 drops Sandalwood, 2 drops Vanilla, and 1 drop Jasmine or Ylang in your diffuser.

Place the mood For An Intimate Dinner with this diffuser blend from Birch Hill Happenings by combining 2 drops each of Black Pepper, Grapefruit, and Jasmine essential oils. "It will establish the evenings feeling for what lies ahead!"

4. Holiday Celebration Essential Oil Blends

Odor Web provides an excellent Essential Oil Recipe for Celebrating, Giving Thanks and Expressing Gratitude using Grapefruit, Bergamot, Frankincense, Cypress and Ginger. "Combine all oils in a clean glass bottle and diffuse as you'd other essential oil combines as you give thanks, pray or meditate."

To warm up the atmosphere in your house this holiday season, try the Cinnamon Spice Diffuser Blend of 2 – 4 drops Cinnamon, 4 – 6 drops Patchouli, 1 – 2 drops Clove, 3 – 5 drops Sweet Orange.

Laura on Green Dwelling Ladies proposes two great combinations for party of the holidays. Fall In Love With Fall by combining 4 drops each of Wild Orange and Cassia essential oils.

Or mix up some Holiday Bliss with Laura's combination of TWO drops each White Fir, Cassia, and Wild Orange essential oils.

5. Essential Oil Insect Repellent Blends

This insect-repelling mixture from Easy Aromatherapy Recipes may also help to cool you back on a hot summer day. Diffuse a mixture of 4 – 6 drops Spearmint, 3 – 5 drops Peppermint, 3 – 5 drops Citronella, and 1 drop Lemongrass essential oils.

6. Essential Oil Combinations for Strain Relief

When you have that stressed feeling, Aroma Web proposes these 4 diffuser blends using the soothing power of Clary Sage, Lavender, Vetiver, Flowery oils and Citrus.

Take this advantage away with this Quieting Diffuser Combination from Birch Hill Happenings.

"It's a nice aromatherapy diffuser essential oil for guys (with the palmarosa) because it's not overly girly. Including a drop of vetiver will give this recipe a smoky undertone."

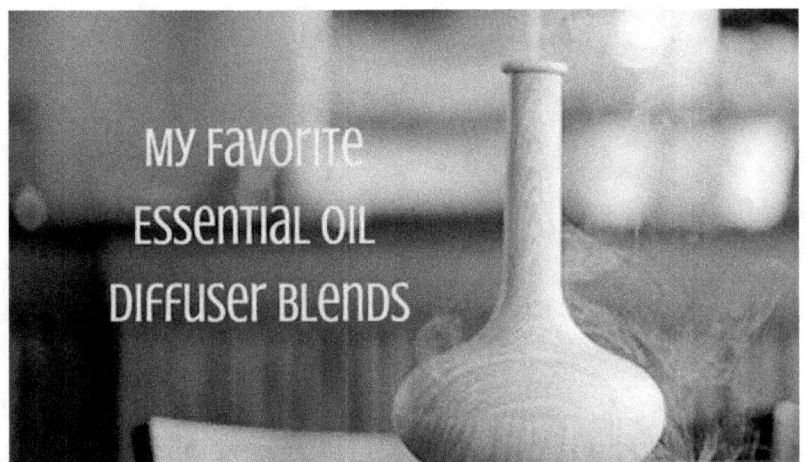

My Favorite
Essential Oil
Diffuser Blends

For anxiety relief, Laura on Green Living Women recommends her Still Diffusing Blend of 3 drops each of Lavender, Geranium, and Roman Chamomile, plus two drops each of Clary Sage and Ylang essential oils.

7. Mood-Lifting Essential Oil Blends

Aroma Web proposes 4 mood-lifting recipes using Sandalwood, Clary Sage, Lavender, together with several Citrus and Floral oils. "These recipes may help during times of depression and anxiety."

To produce a great feeling when friends, as well as family, are gathered together, try this Entertaining Blend from Birch Hill Happenings by combining 3 drops Bergamot, 2 drops Geranium and 3 drops Lavender essential oils in your diffuser.

For a quick pick-me-up, Laura on Green Living Women urges diffusing Be Joyful, a combination of equal parts citrus oil blend including Eden's Garden Simply Citrus or do TERRA Citrus Bliss plus a mood-lifting oil mix like Eden's Garden Joy or do TERRA Elevation.

8. Essential Oil Combinations for Resistance Support

During the spring and summer months, Jill of The Prairie Homestead suggests diffusing two drops each of Lavender, Lemon, and Peppermint essential oils "to keep clear breathing along with a healthy immune response."

To fortify respiratory function during cold and flu season, Jill additionally urges blending one drop each of Peppermint, Lemon, Lime, Eucalyptus and Rosemary essential oils.

When you feel a bug coming on, add several drops to your diffuser to assist your body to fight it fast!

"This fusion should be diffused throughout the cold and flu season."

9. LET'S FOCUS ESSENTIAL OIL DIFFUSER RECIPE

This really is a much-loved combo, and for good cause! It's perfect to increase alertness, or when you are in need of a fast pick-me-up.

2 drops essential oil wild orange

2 drops peppermint essential oil

10.   FRESH AND CLEAN ESSENTIAL OIL DIFFUSER RECIPE

This blend is excellent for creating a welcoming atmosphere at home. It's vivid and fresh:

2 drops lemon essential oil

2 drops rosemary essential oil

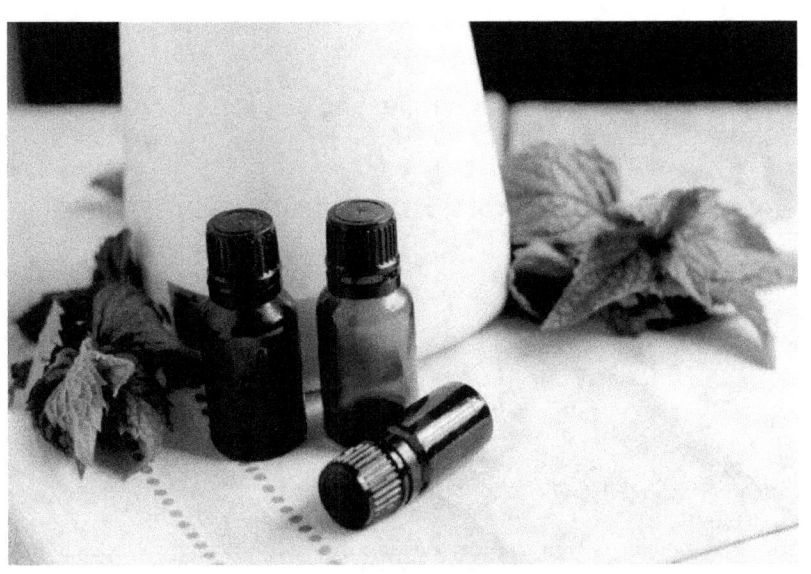

Chapter 2 – Spring Diffuser Recipes and Blends 11 to 20

11. ESSENTIAL OIL ODOR ELIMINATOR DIFFUSER RECIPE

2 drops lemon essential oil

1-drop Melaleuca essential oil

1-drop cilantro essential oil

1-drop lime essential oil

12. ESSENTIAL OIL SEASONAL SUPPORT DIFFUSER RECIPE

These three oils collectively are breathtaking for helping maintain clear breathing and also a healthy immune response. I use this combination, especially during the spring and summer months.

2 drops essential oil lavender

2 drops lemon essential oil

2 drops peppermint essential oil

13. CITRUS EXPLOSION ESSENTIAL OIL DIFFUSER RECIPE

1 drops lemon essential oil

2 drops essential oil wild orange

1-drop lime essential oil

1-drop grapefruit essential oil

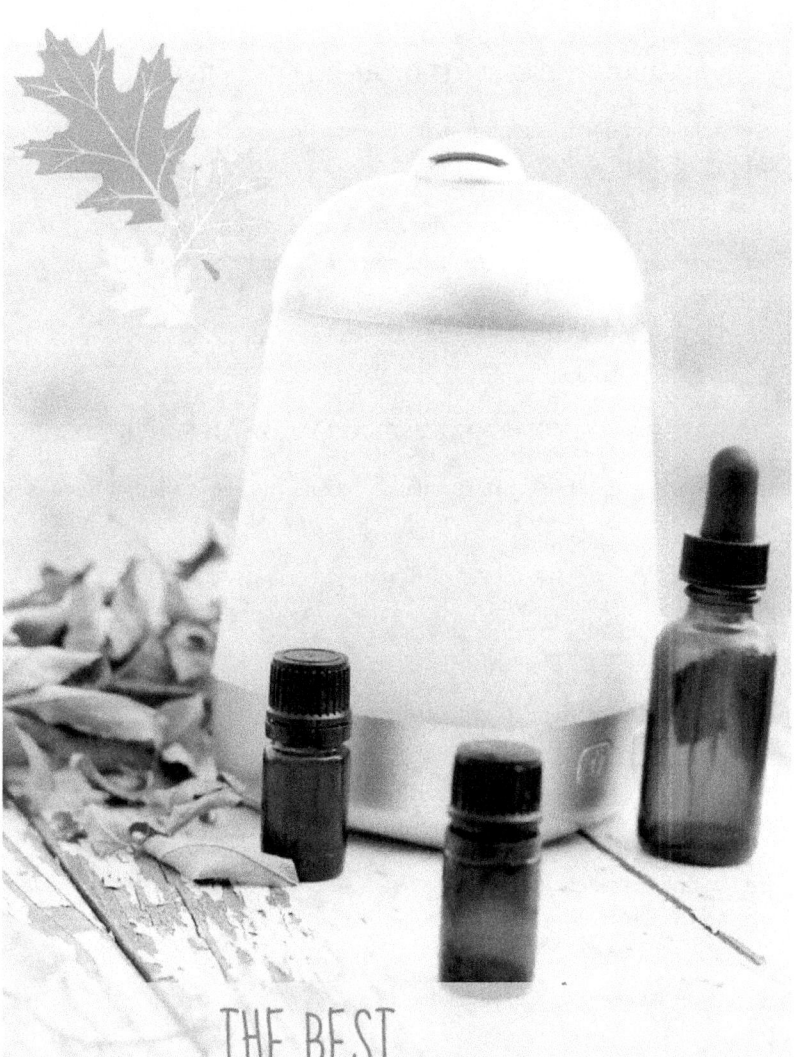

THE BEST
ESSENTIAL OIL DIFFUSER
RECIPES FOR FALL

14. DEEP BREATHE ESSENTIAL OIL DIFFUSER RECIPE

I tend to be a very high-energy person. The good part of that? The awful part? I have difficulty settling down sometimes.

I adore this combination for the evenings when I'm attempting to slow my brain down, and I also like to diffuse it in the bedroom as I fall asleep:

1-drop bergamot essential oil

1-drop patchouli essential oil

15. RESPIRATORY SUPPORT ESSENTIAL OIL DIFFUSER RECIPE

Use this mix to support respiratory function—notably during the winter months.

1 drops lemon essential oil

1-drop eucalyptus essential oil

2 drops peppermint essential oil

1-drop rosemary essential oil

16. FLOWER GARDEN ESSENTIAL OIL DIFFUSER RECIPE

Need your house to smell like a flower garden in full bloom? Try this one:

1 drop geranium essential oil

2 drops essential oil lavender

2 drops roman chamomile essential oil

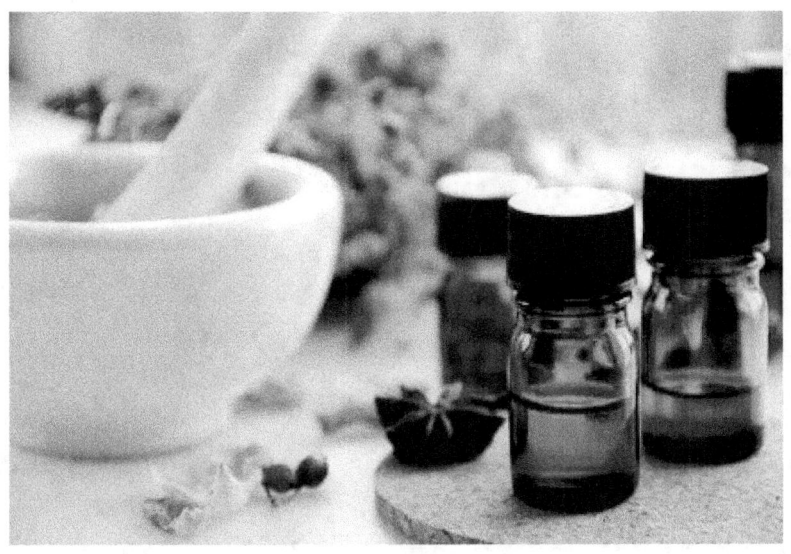

17. MAN-CAVE ESSENTIAL OIL DIFFUSER RECIPE

I believe this combo smells very masculine and woodsy... Although I love it too.

2 drops white first essential oil

2 drops cypress essential oil

2 drops wintergreen essential oil

18. ESSENTIAL OIL BUG REPELLENT DIFFUSER RECIPE

1-drop lemongrass essential oil

1-drop thyme essential oil

1-drop eucalyptus essential oil

1-drop basil essential oil

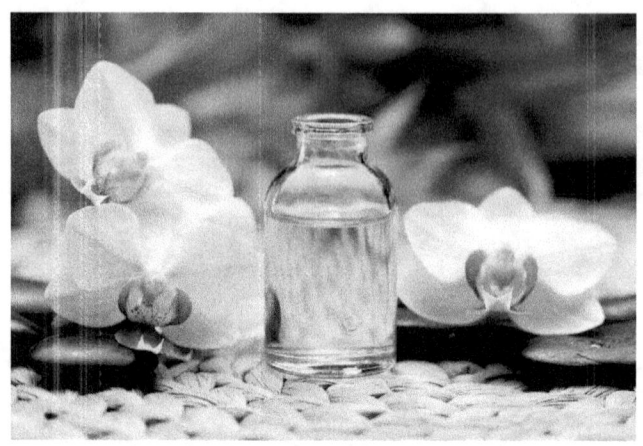

19. ESSENTIAL OIL SPICED CHAI DIFFUSER RECIPE

Craving a cup of chai? Either chai tea homemade concentrate, or put this combination in your diffuser:

2 drops cassia essential oil

3 drops cardamom essential oil

1 drop ginger essential oil

2 drops clove essential oil

20.   WOODSY ESSENTIAL OIL DIFFUSER RECIPE

3 drops essential oil frankincense

2 drops essential oil white fir

1-drop essential oil cedar wood

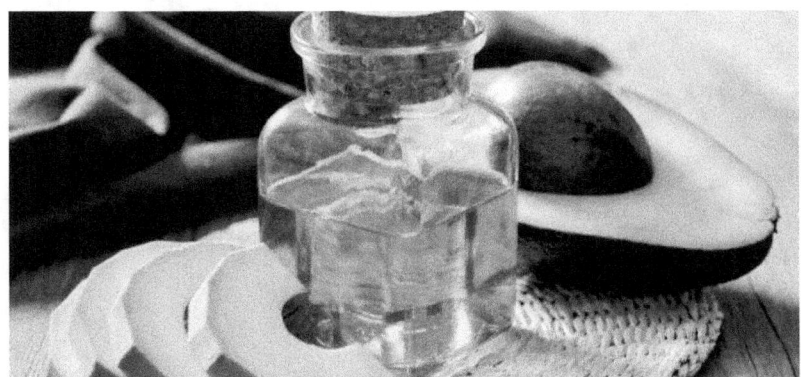

Chapter 3 – Spring Diffuser Recipes and Blends 21 to 30

21.   ESSENTIAL OIL IMMUNE BOOSTER DIFFUSER RECIPE

One of my favorite combinations for the autumn and winter months:

1-drop rosemary essential oil

One drop clove essential oil

1-drop eucalyptus essential oil

1-drop cinnamon barks essential oil

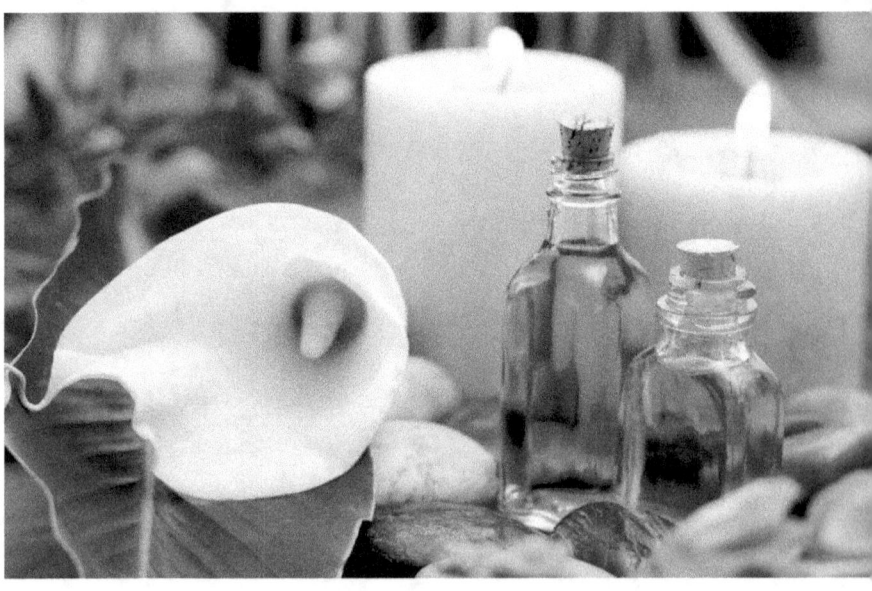

22.   ESSENTIAL OIL G'NIGHT DIFFUSER RECIPE

For a pleasant night's slumber:

2 drops essential oil lavender

2 drops chamomile essential oil

2 drops vetiver essential oil

(For an essential oils for better slumber, click HERE)

23.   CANDY STORE ESSENTIAL OIL DIFFUSER RECIPE

I don't understand why, but this one smells like sweet. The kids adore it, and it'll make your house happy.

Two drop wintergreen essential oil

24.   ENERGIZE ESSENTIAL OIL DIFFUSER RECIPE

2 drops essential oil wild orange

2 drops essential oil frankincense

2 drops cinnamon essential oil

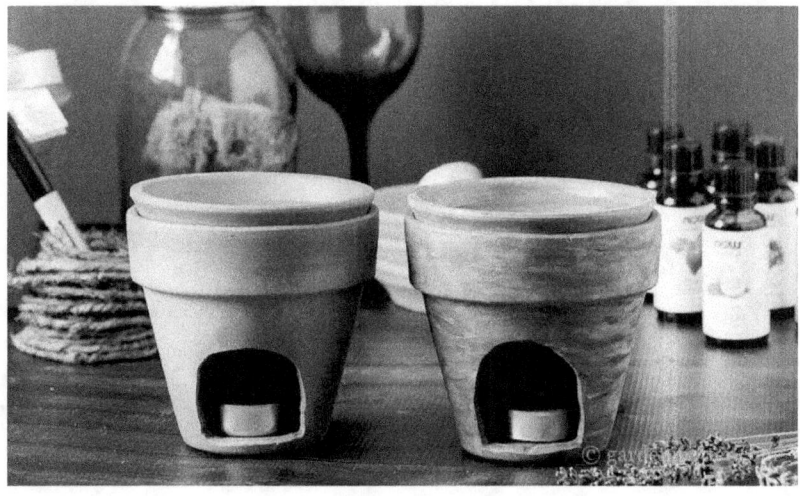

25.   ESSENTIAL OIL GROUNDING DIFFUSER RECIPE

For those moments when everyone has to chill out:

2 drops Vetiver essential oil

2 drops essential oil cedarwood

26.   MUST ATTEMPT ESSENTIAL OIL MIXTURES TO UTILIZE IN YOUR DIFFUSER

Diffusing oil is a good method to not only make your house smell wonderful and clean your atmosphere but has many proven health benefits along with being a proven solution to assist your body to relax. For those who have been using essential oils for some time or whether you're totally new to diffusing I trust you can discover some amazing new uses for your oils. Here are a few of my most favorite MUST ATTEMPT essential oil combinations to utilize in your diffuser.

27.   MY FAVOURITE ESSENTIAL OIL BLENDS:

Relaxing: My husband adores the woodsy aroma of this one!

Energizing: Add 4 drops of peppermint and 4 of citrus fresh.

Simply because: I truly adore grapefruit and peppermint on a regular basis.

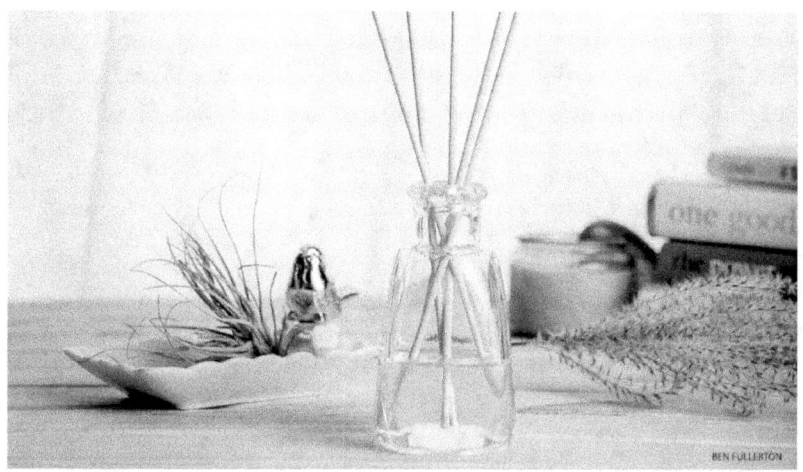

BEN FULLERTON

28. ESSENTIAL OIL BLENDS FOR A RESTFUL SLEEP:

This incorporation has a light scent and is excellent to make use of while winding down at the close of the day.

Goodnight Sleep Mix:

Essential Oil Diffuser

29. ESSENTIAL OIL BLENDS FOR IMMUNE SUPPORT:

Feel Better Mix: Attempt diffusing this one through cold and flu season!

Allergy Alleviation Mix: Add 4 drops of Lavender oil and 4 drops of Peppermint oil in your diffuser and allow it to run. It is an excellent approach to get relief from allergies when you are sleeping. Also it'll clean the atmosphere reducing pollen and other allergens.

30. PEPPERMINT ESSENTIAL OIL USES:

Enhance Attention During Assignments Time – Attempt diffusing peppermint during your kid's assignments time to encourage better focus.

Vacation Scented Ornaments Salt Dough – Peppermint is an ideal aroma for the holidays, so ensure that you add some peppermint essential oil to your salt dough mix before making some Peppermint Scented Candy Cane Decorations with the children!

Add some peppermint to this simple homemade play dough recipe for some gay and invigorating sensory play.

Make some peppermint-scented rice for some fun vacation sensory play.

Dilute nicely with a carrier oil (we use coconut oil) and run on a kid's torso to encourage better breathing when they have a cold.

Chapter 4 – Spring Diffuser Recipes and Blends 31 to 40

31. LEMON ESSENTIAL OIL USES:

Child-Made Energizing Sugar Scrub – Get the children to help make this Energizing Lemon Sugar Scrub as a present for their teachers (or YOU!).

Clean Children Toys – Use lemon in this substance-free soak to wash children toys.

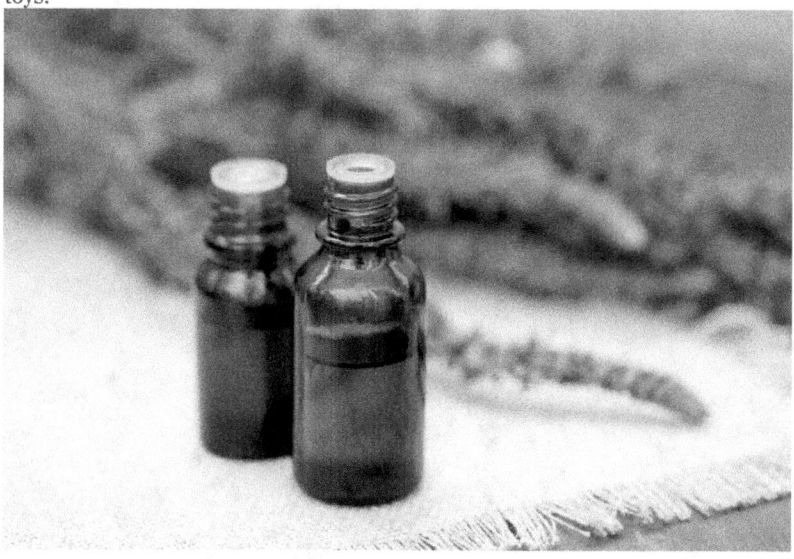

32. LAVENDER ESSENTIAL OIL USES:

Before-Bed Lavender Play dough – Add several drops of lavender essential oil to some homemade play dough for the best kid-still before-bed sensory play.

Take a look at these 4 methods you may safely use lavender essential oil to calm a fussy baby.

Child-Made Still Sugar Scrub – Have the children help make this Lavender Calming Sugar Scrub for a present for their teacher or grandmother.

Child-Calming Bath Bombs – Whip up some lavender bath bombs to toss in the youngster's bedtime bath to encourage calming and better sleep.

Scatter Lavender on Pillows – Scatter a drop or two of lavender on the children' (and YOUR) pillows before bed to support relaxation and better sleep.

Have some homemade lavender cloud dough prepared in a bin for some calming afterschool sensory play?

Soothe Mild Burns – Use a couple of drops of lavender essential oil to slight burns to encourage healing.

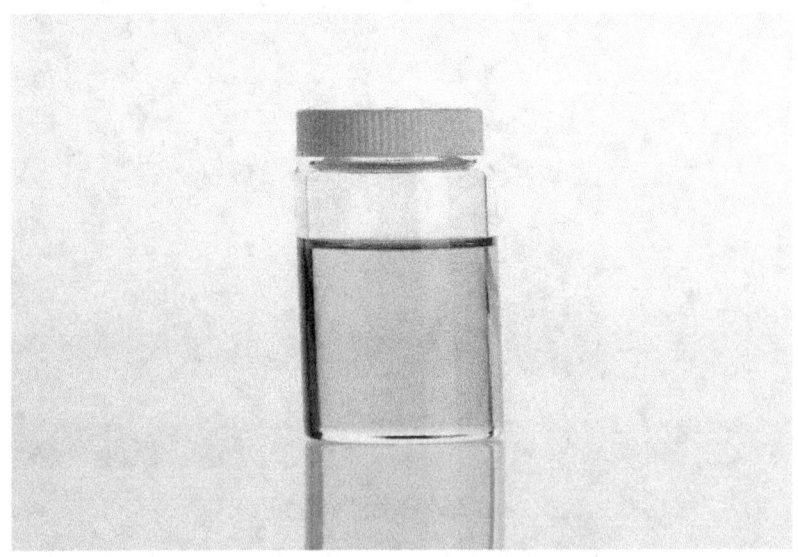

33.   CITRUS FRESH ESSENTIAL OIL MIX USES:

Citrus-Scented Homemade Playdough – Turn homemade play dough sensory play into an experience mood-boosting with the addition of a couple of globules of Citrus Fresh or Lemon essential oils.

34.   FRANKINCENSE ESSENTIAL OIL USES:

Add some Frankincense to a carrier oil to massage on extending pregnancy abdomen skin.

Foster Mama's Immune System when everyone's Ill – Attempt this Immune Fostering Tea recipe that uses frankincense together with lemon and peppermint oils to enhance resistance when the remainder of the family is ill.

Child-Made Lotion Present – Have the children help make some skin-nourishing lotion presents using frankincense and lavender for a kind teacher present.

Support Meditation & Prayer – Diffuse frankincense if you want to support a meditative or prayerful setting.

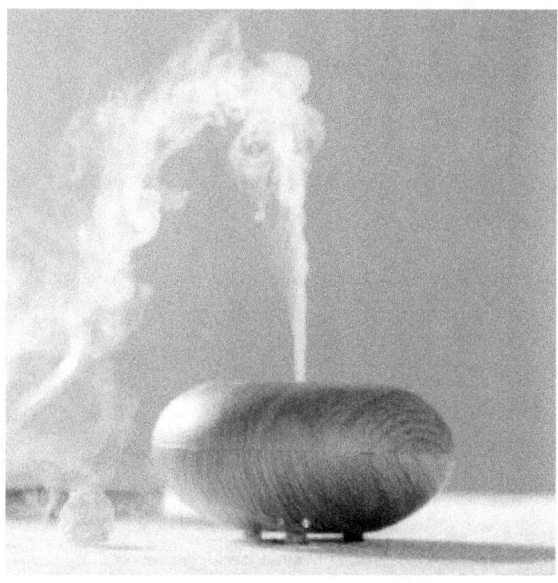

35.   PANAWAY ESSENTIAL OIL MIX USES:

Relieve Pregnancy Muscle Aches & Pains

Soothe Tired & Raw Mama Feet

36.   TEA TREE ESSENTIAL OIL USES:

Natural Homemade Diaper Wipes – This recipe for homemade diaper wipes joins tea tree oil and lavender oil to soothe and clean infant's underside.

Dab on Skin Scrapes –

Home Made (Insect Repellent) Hair Detangler –

Soothe Dry Skin –

Homemade Laundry Detergent – Join tea tree oil with lavender, thieves, and a few other ingredients to produce your laundry detergent!

37.   ROBBERS ESSENTIAL OIL MIX USES:

Ill-Day Slime – Add a few robbers to a homemade slime recipe to produce the best resistance-boosting sensory play action for a sick day.

Diffuse During Flu Season – Keep the robbers going in the diffuser throughout flu season to improve the family's immune systems. (A diffuser comes with all the Young Living Premium Kit!)

Rub on Ill Children' Feet – Dilute robbers with some carrier oil (we use coconut oil) and rub it on your ill children' feet to foster their immune systems.

Soothe Teething Gums –

Child-Safe Surface Cleanser – Add 10 drops of robbers and ONE teaspoon.

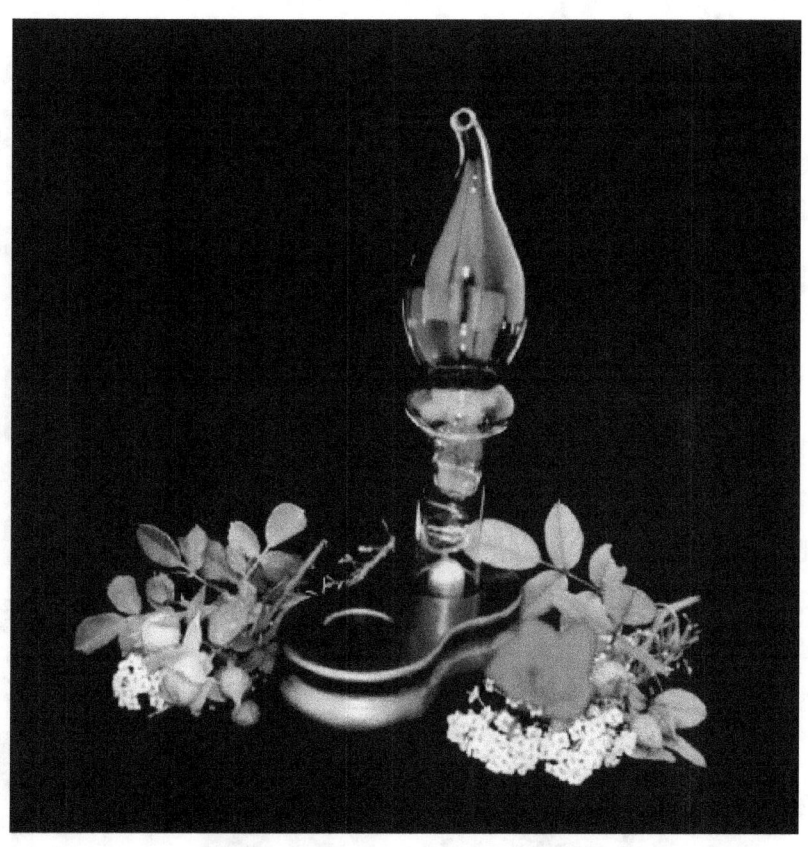

38.   STRESS AWAY ESSENTIAL OIL COMBINATION USES:

Calm and Concerned Kid – Place a couple of drops of tension away behind the ears of your nervous child before they head off to school.

Mood-Boosting Bubble Bath – Use pressure away in this homemade bubble bath recipe to improve your kid's mood with a straightforward bath.

39.   PLEASURE ESSENTIAL OIL BLEND USES:

Perfume for an Exhausted Mama – Boost your mood (and encourage a little romance!) as the end of a tiring day by dabbing a couple of drops of joy on your wrists and neck.

Diffuse During an At Home Date Night – Put a few globules of happiness in the diffuser after the kids go to bed to inspire love affair for an at-home date night. (A diffuser comes with all the Young Living Premium Kit!)

Chemical-Free Child Cologne – Dab some drops of Delight in your little girl's wrists for her to wear cologne like mama.

Diffuse During Mama Time – Add some pleasure to your diffuser when you have a few kid-free minutes to enhance your mood.

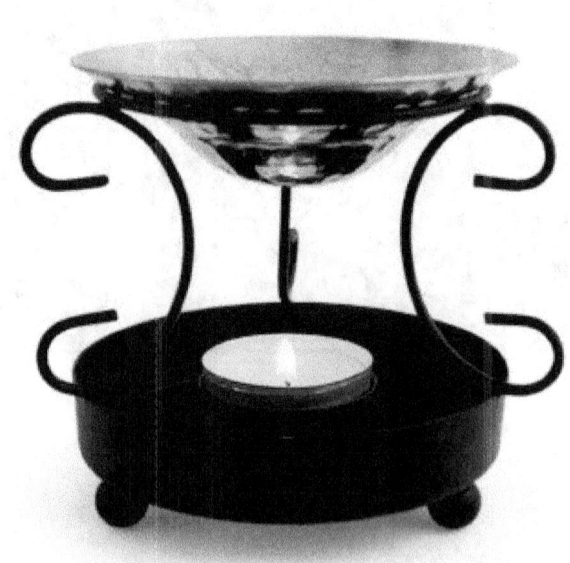

40.   PURIFICATION ESSENTIAL OIL MIX USES:

Apply to Insect Bites – Apply a drop of Purification to the children' bug bites to soothe them and promote healing.

Help with Diaper Odors – Throw a cotton ball with a couple of globules of purification into the diaper bin to help eliminate the odors.

Eliminate Odors Diffuse to Help – To your diffuser Add purification after the kids have gotten ill (on the carpet...) to help purify the air and remove odors. (A diffuser comes with the Young Living Premium Kit!)

Help for Stinky Shoes – Add a few globules of purification to cotton balls into the shoes of your kids. Leave overnight to help remove the scent.

An Essential Oil Reference Book – It will either be the Essentials Oils Reference Guide.

The Essential Oil Starter Guide – a gorgeous 20-page booklet that covers uses for every one of the essential oils in the starter set.

Chapter 5 – Spring Diffuser Recipes and Blends 41 to 50

41. Muscle Pain:

2 drops Lavender

Add 2 drops lavender and 2 drops rosemary oil to 4 teaspoons of our massage oil base (or some plain base/carrier oil).

Headaches:

2 drops Lavender

Massage 2 drops undiluted lavender into the temples as well as the base of the skull.

Pre-Sports Rub:

2 drops Rosemary

1 drops Lavender

1 drops Eucalyptus

First, mix all the essential oils together, and then add to 4 teaspoons of our massage oil base (or some plain base/carrier oil). And then gently mix them all together.

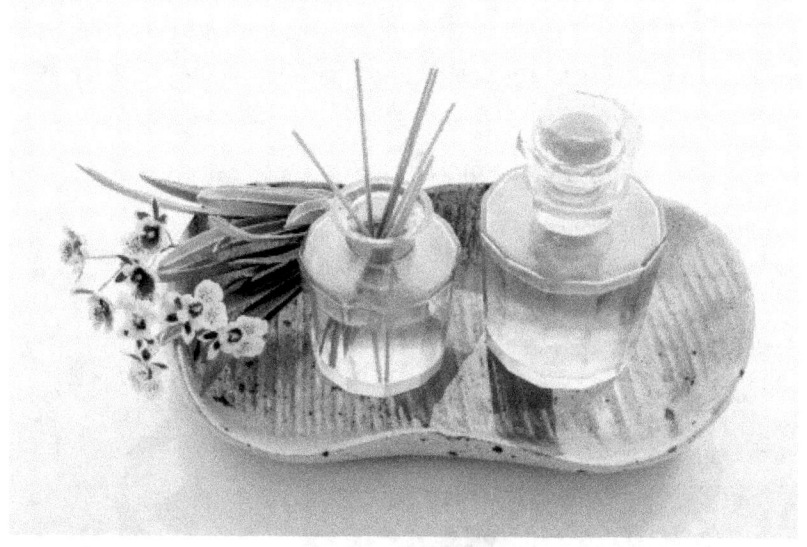

42. Relaxing Aromatherapy Blends:

Relaxation Massage Oil

4 drops Lavender

1 drop Petitgrain

1 drop Frankincense

Add the above-mentioned essential oil to 6 teaspoon of massage base. Add to a warm bath or use for a relaxing massage blend.

To Calm Nerves and Encourage Slumber:

4 drops Lavender

Add 4 drops lavender to a teaspoon of milk or cream. Decant into a warm bath, stir bathwater and soak.

Or

Add 4 drops lavender to 4 teaspoons of our massage oil base (or some plain base/carrier oil). The area in a diffuser and diffuse into your room.

43.   Uplifting Aromatherapy Recipes

Uplifting Personal Blend for Daytime Use:

2 drops Geranium

2 drops Rosewood

2 drops Bergamot

Wear as a scent, use for a gentle massage or inhale right from the bottle.

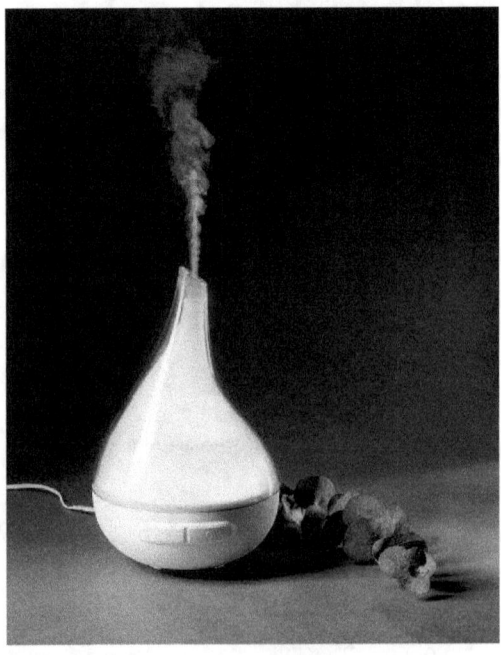

44.   Uplifting Personal Blend for Nighttime Use:

2 drops HoWood

2 drops Bergamot

Add 1-drop howood, two drops Bergamot and two drops ylang ylang to 6 teaspoons of our massage oil base (or any plain base/carrier oil). Wear as a fragrance, use as a massage blend or inhale right from the bottle.

45.   Sparkling Candy Cane

This mix is wonderfully lovely (although not very so) and extremely reminiscent of Holiday candy canes because of the peppermint acrylic. The vanilla offers this mixture a subtle warmth and sweetness that gives it together.

Add to your diffuser:

• Distilled water

• 8 drops peppermint essential oil

• 2 drops vanilla essential oil

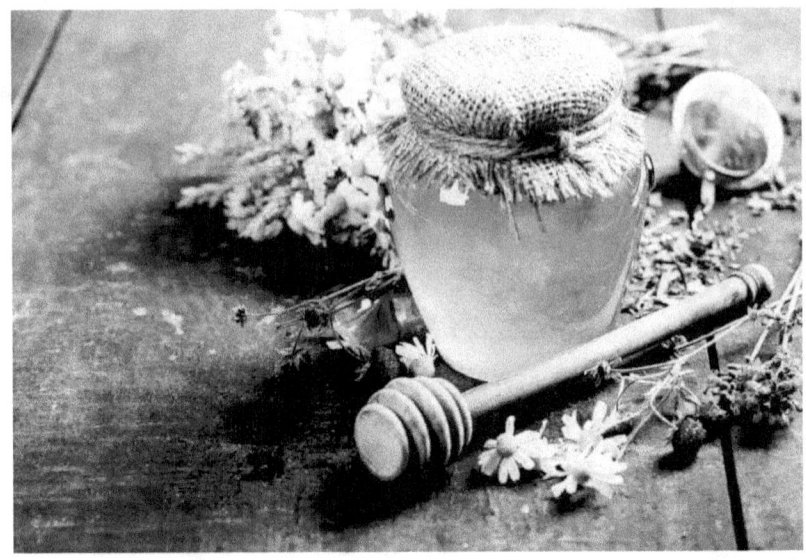

46.   Mulled Cider

This is a great blend to diffuse while snuggled up nearby the fire having a good book and a hot mug of cider. The citrusy notes get this to mix shiny and appealing for almost any holiday occasion.

Enhance your diffuser:

• 4 drops orange gas

• 2 drops nutmeg gas

• One drop of clove essential oil

47.   Spiced Cider

This blend has a spicier note compared to the mulled cider mixture, hence the title. The ginger and cinnamon essential oils provide warmth as the red sweetens the recipe.

Increase your diffuser:

• Distilled water

• 4 drops orange gas

• 3 drops oil of cinnamon bark essential

• 3 drops ginger essential oil

48.   Pumpkin Pie

Who doesn't appreciate the fragrance of freshly cooked pumpkin pie? This mixture fills your house with a delicious smell that will make guests wonder what smells so incredible! It's a perfect Holiday scent that gets everyone into Christmas cheer.

Add to your diffuser:

• Distilled water

• 2 drops cardamom gas

• 2 drops oil of cinnamon bark essential

• 3 drops nutmeg gas

• 2 drops ginger gas

• 1-drop vanilla acrylic

49.   Snickerdoodle Cookie

The odor of freshly baked cookies is intoxicating and what's fantastic about that recipe is you don't need to be baking as a way to relish it for unlimited hours. This mix severely smells JUST like snickerdoodle cookies, and it is one of my personal favorite diffuser blends for Christmas today.

Increase your diffuser:

• Distilled water

• 5 drops orange essential oil

• One drop clove gas

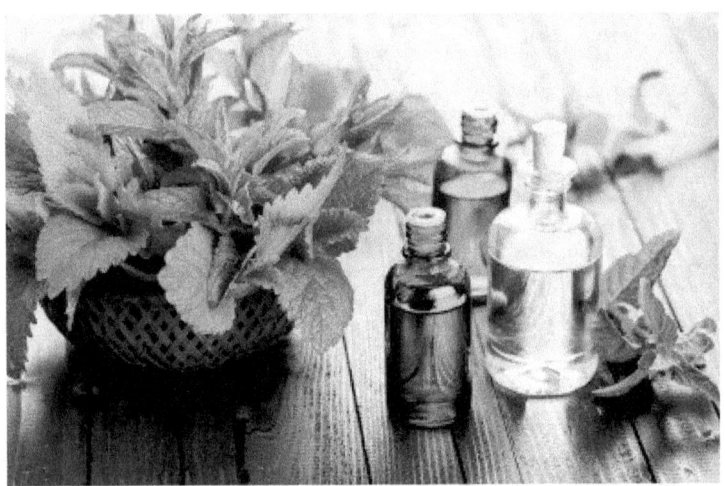

50. Winter Wonderland

If you love the aroma of pine, then this can be a great combination to soften. My fiancé LOVES this blend before bedtime since they can imagine being out in the wilderness. I find that most men like this formula.

Enhance your diffuser:

• Three drops balsam fir essential oil

• Two drops Spruce gas

• 2 drops peppermint essential oil

- One drop juniper essential oil

Chapter 6- Tips to Clean Your Home With Essential Oils

Here's without the stress of substances, fumes, or synthetics harming our bodies, where we can change to a brand new concept of cleaning. Essential oils would be the best-kept secret for purifying and cleaning your environment.

Surprisingly, essential oils are just as strong as traditional cleaners.

It's a great deal less expensive and quite simple when you use essential oils instead of store bought routine cleaners. The essential oils in this post antibacterial, antiviral, anti-fungal and anti-microbial. And the best part is they're even good and 100% safe for you! Cleaners that are normal can't say that.

Using the highest quality therapeutic grade essential oils (like Young Living's) is of extreme importance. Inferior quality oils aren't effective in killing germs, nor are they safe to utilize in the ways.

Here are some strategies to attain a healthy, clean dwelling using essential oils.

Floorings:

If you mop your floors

(tile, wood, laminate, marble) - replace your floor cleaner and make use of a pail of water with 10-20 drops of Lemon and/or Lavender essential oils. Research has provided evidence for that lemon and lavender essential oils kill many strains of bacteria. Plus walk and it's totally safe to inhale upon!

If Roomba your floorings or you steam

(tile, wood, laminate, marble) - walk through the house and drop several globules of Lemon and/or Lavender essential oils in several locations. Especially garbage, by the front door can area, kitchen and toilets. As you steam the flooring, the steamer or room, killing bacteria, mold and viruses will disperse the essential oils in the procedure.

If you vacuum your floors

- Place five drops of Lemon and Lavender essential oil on a tissue and vacuum it up. This may kill the germs that get sucked up into your vacuum and also diffuse the oils into your house leaving it smelling wonderful!

Air Purifiers:

To have a clean air environment, dispose of that air freshener that is plugged into your wall! Its fragrance is certainly not of curative worth. Use a couple of drops of Robbers or essential oil blends that are Purification on a cotton ball and place it in your AC vent. Both of those mixes were formulated to kill viruses, airborne bacteria, mold and fungus. In addition, they neutralize smoke and pet odors.

Or better yet, obtain a cold air diffuser and diffuse either of the essential oils every day.

Hand Wash:

To make a chemical free, germ-killing hand wash, use the rest of your foaming hand save and wash the bottle up. Fill the rest with spring water. Add ten drops of Thieves essential oil. Shake well and use the kitchen as well as bathroom sinks.

Hand Disinfectant:

Loosened your Purell and get a bottle of Lemon essential oil. Rub 1 drop of Lemon essential oil into hands after using public restrooms.

See how only a few changes in your cleaning routine can certainly replace a lot of chemical cleaning products in your home? I suggest beginning slow by removing one cleaning product per week and including an essential oil in its area. Shortly you will be actual "greener" than anyone else you know and probably a bit fitter, too!

Conclusion

A common ingredient in natural products, essential oils are normally used through inhalation or by external application of diluted oil. Because these oils are so easily accessible to the general public, a lot of people wrongly assume that no special knowledge or training is required to make use of them. Sadly, there are many who make this error. Some have read a little about aromatherapy, or a close friend or provider has told them unique oil is great for this or that.

Some have read a little about aromatherapy, or a friend or provider has told them particular oil is great for this or that. But essential oils can cause problems if used incorrectly.

Plants, which are too delicate for, steam distillation, like jasmine, orange blossom, and rose, can have their oils extracted using solvents. Oils created by this process are called absolutes and are used in perfumes or diffusers because the solvent deposit makes most of them unsuitable for external use.

The system of generation is just one factor affecting the product quality and price of these botanical extracts. Others include the rarity of the plant, how and where it had been grown, how many plants are essential to make the oil, as well as the quality standards of the maker. Genuine rose oil, for example, is not exceptionally cheap. This can be mere as it requires 200 pounds of roses (around 60,000 blossoms) to make 1 ounce of rose oil. That equals 30 roses to get a single drop! In the event you are paying less than $80 for a 5-milliliter bottle of rose oil, it is either synthetic, or it has been diluted using a carrier oil for example jojoba. Purchasing diluted oil is totally okay as long as you know what you are getting. Reputable suppliers will be up front about whether their products can be purchased already diluted. Less reputable suppliers may be selling an adulterated incorporation (for instance, a touch of rose oil mixed with more affordable rose geranium oil) and asserting it is 100 percent rose oil.

These are all mixed artificial scents that might additionally include phthalates as well as other possibly hazardous ingredients and are diluted with propylene glycol, mineral oil, or vegetable oil. Synthetics are not a lot more expensive than essential oils, as well as their smell is quite a bit stronger. When you will smell the candles from the exterior and walk past a candle store, that's artificial scent. So-called essential oils promoted under these names are almost always artificial.

In case you would like to make use of essential oils, it's critically crucial that you think of these like another recovering tool: get appropriate training within their use, completely research contraindications and interactions. Like other things that may be placed on the body, essential oils could cause injury. Recall, "natural" doesn't automatically mean an item is mild or safe. There are oils that should never be utilized on a person who has high blood pressure and oils that interact with specific drugs. Cypress and rosemary can be dangerous if a female is pregnant or nursing. And some essential oils, like wintergreen, can even be fatal if ingested.

FREE Bonus Reminder

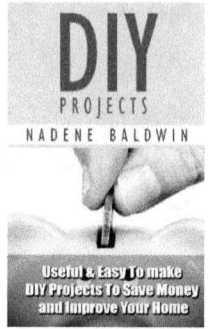

If you have not grabbed it yet, please go ahead and download your special bonus report *"DIY Projects. 13 Useful & Easy To Make DIY Projects To Save Money & Improve Your Home!"*

Simply Click the Button Below

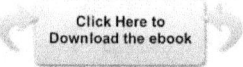

OR **Go to This Page**

http://diyhomecraft.com/free

BONUS #2: More Free & Discounted Books

Do you want to receive more Free & Discounted Books?

We have a mailing list where we send out our new Books when they go free or with a discount on Kindle. Click on the link below to sign up for Free & Discount Book Promotions.

=> Sign Up for Free & Discount Book Promotions <=

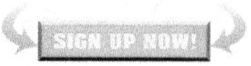

OR Go to this URL

http://zbit.ly/1WBb1Ek

www.ingramcontent.com/pod-product-compliance
Lightning Source LLC
Chambersburg PA
CBHW061802280526
45787CB00003BA/1449